LOWER YOUR BLOOD PRESSURE NATURALLY

Fruits That Minimize Blood Pressure And Heart Health

ASHLEY GREY

TABLE OF CONTENT

INTRODUCTION

The increased prevalence of high blood pressure is becoming a matter of concern in the fast-paced world of today. If left untreated, the so-called silent killer can cause serious health problems. The good news is that nature has given us a wealth of resources to properly address this health problem. We will examine the revolutionary potential of fruits and herbal teas to lower high blood pressure and improve heart health in general in this extensive guide.

The management of hypertension by modern medicine has come a long way, yet natural therapies are still quite important. Fruits are critical for cardiovascular health since they are a great source of vital vitamins, minerals, and antioxidants. Similar to this, natural teas made from plants and herbs have been prized for their therapeutic qualities for millennia in a wide range of civilizations. They work together to create a powerful alliance in the pursuit of heart health.

We will take a trip through the vibrant world of fruits in the upcoming chapters, learning about their special qualities and creative ways to include them in your regular diet. Every fruit, from the subtle sweetness of berries to the tangy enticement of citrus fruits, offers a variety of nutrients that can aid in naturally regulating blood pressure in addition to delicious flavors.

In parallel, we will delve into the fragrant world of natural teas and learn about the therapeutic qualities of herbs such as black, green, and hibiscus tea. Perfectly made, these teas provide a variety of heart-healthy components in addition to a reassuring ritual. You'll discover how to choose, brew, and savor these teas to optimize their potency.

Join us on this enlightening journey as we unlock the secrets of lowering blood pressure naturally. By embracing the bounties of nature and incorporating them into your daily routine, you can go on a path toward a healthier heart and a happier life. However, this guide is not just about incorporating fruits and teas into your diet; it's also about understanding the science behind their impact on blood pressure. We will unravel the mysteries of hypertension, exploring the factors that contribute to its rise and the mechanisms through which fruits and natural teas exert their positive influence.

CHAPTER ONE

Orange Juice

Orange juice is a widely used beverage that is appreciated for both its nutritional value and pleasant flavor on a global scale. Orange juice is not a direct blood pressure reducer, but it can be a component of a balanced diet that helps protect the heart.

Oranges are high in antioxidants, potassium, and vitamin C, all of which support cardiovascular health in general. Specifically, potassium is necessary for controlling blood pressure. A diet high in potassium balances salt levels in the body, hence lowering blood pressure. Oranges and their juice are a fantastic option for anyone trying to maintain appropriate blood pressure levels because they are naturally high in potassium and low in salt.

Furthermore, flavonoids, one type of antioxidant present in orange juice, have been connected to better blood vessel health. To keep blood pressure at normal, healthy blood arteries are essential. Research has indicated that eating foods high in flavonoids, such as oranges, may help regulate blood pressure.

Orange juice can be a component of a diet that promotes heart health, but it's crucial to remember that it should only be consumed occasionally. Natural sugars included in orange juice have the potential to increase caloric intake and cause weight gain if ingested in excess. Since being overweight increases the risk of high blood pressure, it's critical to strike a balance between calorie intake and physical exercise.

Because it is devoid of additional sugars and preservatives and keeps more of its natural nutrients, freshly extracted orange juice is preferable to prepackaged juices. Whole oranges are also a wonderful option since they include fiber in the diet, which is good for your digestive system and can help you control your weight.

Although orange juice by itself cannot directly lower blood pressure, it can be a healthy, well-balanced component of a diet that promotes heart health. It's best to speak with a healthcare provider before making any dietary changes, particularly if you have any pre-existing medical disorders or are worried about your blood pressure.

CHAPTER TWO

Lemon Juice

A popular beverage that combines the health benefits of lemons and the refreshing flavor of water is called lemon water. Although it is frequently praised for its possible health advantages, its efficacy as the only treatment for decreasing blood pressure is something that needs to be carefully considered.

Lemons are a great source of vitamin C, which is a potent antioxidant that keeps cells safe from harm and promotes heart health in general. Lemons also contain potassium, a chemical that is essential for controlling blood pressure. Maintaining appropriate blood pressure levels depends on potassium's ability to counteract the effects of sodium in the body.

Lemon juice and water make a tasty, low-calorie beverage that might be a decent substitute for sugar-filled drinks and help with weight management. Sustaining a healthy weight is crucial for blood pressure management since being overweight puts undue strain on the heart and increases the risk of hypertension.

Getting enough water to drink is also essential for good health. Maintaining proper hydration is essential for the body's normal functioning, particularly for the circulatory system, which is crucial for controlling blood pressure. Sufficient hydration promotes healthy blood circulation and preserves the equilibrium of body fluids.

Lemon water should not be seen as a stand-alone treatment for high blood pressure, even though it can be a part of a balanced diet and a healthy lifestyle. A complex disorder, hypertension is impacted by several factors, such as overall lifestyle choices, stress levels, physical activity, food, and heredity.

You must speak with a healthcare provider if your blood pressure worries you. Based on your medical history, they can offer tailored advice and perform the required tests to identify the best course of action. To properly manage high blood pressure, it may occasionally be advised to combine medical therapies with lifestyle alterations such as dietary adjustments, exercise, and stress reduction methods.

Lemon water is not an independent therapy for decreasing blood pressure, but it can help with overall water intake, supply vital minerals, and be a component of a heart-healthy diet. To effectively regulate blood pressure and enhance overall well-being, it is imperative to adopt a holistic approach to health that includes regular exercise, a balanced diet, stress management, and medical supervision when necessary.

CHAPTER THREE

Black Tea

Black tea, which is made from the Camellia plant, is becoming more and more well-known for its possible health advantages, which include lowering blood pressure. Below is a detailed summary of how black tea can be used as a blood pressure remedy:

Vital Elements:

Flavonoids, specifically theaflavins and catechins, are found in black tea. The potential of these antioxidants to lower blood pressure and promote heart health has been investigated.

Blood Pressure Management:

Research indicates that drinking black tea could lower blood pressure a little bit. Black tea's alpha-f may relax blood vessels, improving blood flow and relieving pressure on artery walls.

Qualities of Antioxidants:

Black tea's antioxidants aid in the fight against inflammation and oxidative stress, two conditions that can lead to hypertension. Indirectly, black tea promotes healthy blood pressure levels by lowering these markers.

Production of Nitric Oxide:

It has been discovered that drinking black tea helps the body produce more nitric oxide. By relaxing blood vessels, nitric oxide improves blood circulation and aids in preserving a healthy blood pressure level.

Content of Caffeine:

Although there is some caffeine in black tea, it is not as much as in coffee. Moderate black tea drinking offers a reduced stimulant impact for those who are sensitive to caffeine, potentially preventing excessive excitement and the ensuing rises in blood pressure.

Reduced Stress:

Sipping a cup of tea can be a calming habit. Because stress hormones can elevate blood pressure, reduced stress levels may help lower blood pressure. Black tea helps to maintain healthy blood pressure indirectly by encouraging relaxation.

Hydration

For general health, particularly cardiovascular health, adequate hydration is crucial. Black tea consumption adds to daily fluid consumption and encourages optimal hydration, both of which are necessary for the circulatory system to operate as it should.

Modesty Is Essential:

Although there may be health benefits to black tea, moderation is key when consuming it. Drinking too much tea can result in consuming too much caffeine, which can be harmful to some people.

Speaking with a Medical Professional:

Individuals may react differently to dietary modifications, such as adding black tea. It's best to speak with a healthcare provider before making any big dietary changes, especially if you use medication or have pre-existing medical conditions.

Black tea should be used in moderation and as part of an overall healthy lifestyle. It can support heart health and might help with blood pressure management when included in a balanced diet.

CHAPTER FOUR

Green Tea

One of the many health benefits of green tea that has long been touted is its ability to potentially decrease blood pressure. Hypertension, often known as high blood pressure, is a common medical condition that can have serious side effects like heart disease and stroke. Including green tea in your diet could be a natural remedy for this illness.

Abundant in Antioxidants

Antioxidants found in abundance in green tea, especially catechins, have been shown to improve heart health. These antioxidants aid in the body's defense against dangerous free radicals, lowering oxidative stress and enhancing cardiovascular health in general.

Encourages Leasing:

Green tea contains the amino acid L-theanine, which has relaxing properties for both the body and the mind. It may lessen tension and encourage relaxation, which may obliquely lower blood pressure. Controlling stress is essential for preserving a healthy blood pressure level.

Impacts on the Production of Nitric Oxide:

It has been discovered that the catechins in green tea increase the circulatory system vessels' nitric oxide production. Nitric oxide contributes to blood pressure reduction, improved blood flow, and blood vessel dilatation. Improved control of blood pressure is a result of improved functioning of endothelial cells.

Lowers Cholesterol from LDL:

Taking green tea has been associated with a reduction in low-density lipoprotein (LDL) cholesterol, which is commonly known as "bad" cholesterol. Green tea promotes heart health and can help reduce heart disease by lowering LDL cholesterol levels.

Helps in the Management of Weight:

One important risk factor for hypertension is obesity. Green tea has ingredients that can increase metabolism and help with fat oxidation. Green tea helps to regulate blood pressure indirectly by aiding with weight management.

Enhances Blood Vessel Performance:

Consuming green tea regularly has been linked to enhanced endothelium function, which permits appropriate blood vessel relaxation. Healthy blood pressure levels are maintained in part by this blood vessel relaxation.

Effect of Natural Diuretics:

Due to its modest diuretic properties, green tea helps the body eliminate extra fluid. By doing so, the pressure on the blood vessel walls may be reduced and the amount of blood flowing through the blood vessels may be reduced as well.

Modesty Is Essential:

Even though green tea has several advantages, it's still recommended to drink it in moderation. Too much caffeine, even from green tea, can lead to severe effects. Generally speaking, two to three cups of green tea should be had each day.

It is important to remember that green tea should not be used in place of prescription drugs or medical advice, even if it can be a beneficial complement to a balanced diet. People who have hypertension or any other medical issue should speak with their healthcare practitioner for an accurate diagnosis and advice on how to successfully manage their condition.

CHAPTER FIVE

Tomato Juice

The purported health benefits of tomato juice, such as its capacity to decrease blood pressure, have made it more popular. The consumption of tomato products, especially tomato juice, may help lower blood pressure, according to several studies and research. This is a thorough examination of tomato juice's potential as a blood pressure reducer:

The Composition of Nutrition:

Potassium, vitamins C and E, and antioxidants are just a few of the vital elements found in tomato juice. In particular, potassium is essential for controlling blood pressure because it counteracts the effects of sodium on the body. Consuming a lot of potassium-rich food can aid in blood vessel wall relaxation and lower the risk of hypertension.

Precursors and Lycopene:

Lycopene, a potent antioxidant that gives tomatoes their vivid red color, is found in tomatoes. Numerous health advantages of lycopene have been associated with it, including the possibility of lowering blood pressure. It is thought to lessen oxidative stress and enhance blood vessel function, both of which can raise blood pressure.

Production of Nitric Oxide:

As a result, tomato juice and tomatoes themselves are rich sources of nitrates. Nitric oxide, a substance that helps widen blood vessels and enhance blood flow, is produced by the body from nitrate. Tomato juice helps vasodilation, which in effect can help reduce blood pressure, by increasing the generation of nitric oxide.

Minimal in Sodium and Calories:

In general, tomato juice is low in salt and calories. For people with high blood pressure, a low-sodium diet is advised since too much salt can cause fluid retention and elevated blood pressure. Tomato juice and other low-sodium foods and drinks can be a part of a successful hypertension management plan.

Research Results:

Numerous analyses have looked into the connection between blood pressure and tomato-based goods, such as tomato juice. Research indicates that regular consumption of tomato products can positively affect blood pressure levels, particularly in those with hypertension, but individual reactions may differ.

Method for Including Tomato

Tomato juice is simple to include in your diet. It can be consumed as a cool drink by itself or combined with other vegetable juices to acquire more nutrients. Its flavor can be improved without sacrificing its health benefits by adding herbs and spices. It offers a delicious method to incorporate it into your meals as a foundation for soups and sauces.

Use caution and seek advice:

Tomato juice can be a beneficial supplement to a balanced diet, but it's crucial to remember that everyone reacts differently to different foods. If a person has any allergies or specific medical issues, they should speak with a doctor before making big dietary changes, such as drinking more tomato juice.

While tomato juice by itself might not be a comprehensive approach to controlling high blood pressure, it can undoubtedly be a useful component of a diet that promotes heart health. Tomato juice can help improve blood pressure control and cardiovascular health when paired with a balanced diet, frequent exercise, and an overall healthy lifestyle.

CHAPTER SIX

Hibiscus Tea

The bright and colorful hibiscus plant is used to make hibiscus tea, which has been researched for its possible health advantages, including its potential to decrease blood pressure. Vitamin C, minerals, and antioxidants abound in this herbal tea. According to several studies, drinking hibiscus tea may help reduce hypertension or high blood pressure. Below is a comprehensive summary of its advantages when used as a blood pressure remedy:

Abundant in Antioxidants

Antioxidants found in abundance in hibiscus tea, particularly anthocyanins, aid in the body's fight against oxidative stress. These antioxidants lower the risk of hypertension and enhance heart health generally.

Organic Diuretic Characteristics:

As a natural diuretic, hibiscus tea helps the body flush out excess salt. Lowering sodium levels causes blood arteries to relax, which lowers blood pressure.

Having an impact on ACE (angiotensin-converting enzyme) inhibitors:

Hibiscus tea may function similarly to ACE inhibitors, a family of drugs that are frequently used for hypertension, according to some studies. ACE inhibitors reduce blood pressure by preventing the synthesis of an enzyme that narrows blood vessels, hence relaxing blood vessels.

Reduces LDL Cholesterol

High LDL cholesterol can cause artery plaque to accumulate, raising blood pressure. Lower LDL cholesterol levels have been demonstrated to improve heart health when hibiscus tea is consumed.

Lowers Levels of Blood Sugar:

The anti-diabetic qualities of hibiscus tea may aid in lowering blood sugar levels. As hypertension can be exacerbated by high blood sugar, controlling diabetes well can help lower blood pressure.

Unwinding and Decreased Stress:

Hibiscus tea's relaxing properties can aid in lowering tension and anxiety. Maintaining appropriate blood pressure levels requires finding strategies to de-stress and relax because long-term stress can exacerbate hypertension.

Enhances Endothelial Performance:

The inner lining of blood arteries is called the endothelium. It has been discovered that hibiscus tea enhances endothelial function, improving the blood vessels' capacity to dilate and maintain appropriate blood flow—a critical role in blood pressure regulation.

Precautions and Dosage:

Despite the possible health benefits of hibiscus tea, you should always speak with a doctor before using it, particularly if you already use blood pressure medication. They can keep an eye on your development and offer you advice on the proper dosage.

Because of its many health benefits and its natural chemical makeup, hibiscus tea is a promising blood pressure-lowering treatment. However, it is important to regard its use as an adjunct to a healthy lifestyle, which includes stress reduction, regular exercise, and a balanced diet—all of which are critical for maintaining ideal blood pressure levels.

CHAPTER SEVEN

Juice of Pomegranates

Pomegranate juice's possible health benefits—particularly about heart health and blood pressure regulation—have drawn a lot of attention in recent years. Pomegranate juice is a well-liked natural treatment for hypertension as several research indicate that it may help lower blood pressure.

Abundant in Antioxidants

Antioxidants abound in pomegranate juice, including flavonoids, anthocyanins, and toxins. By lowering stress and preventing oxidative stress, these antioxidants support better cardiovascular health.

Production of Nitric Oxide:

It has been demonstrated that pomegranate juice increases the body's synthesis of nitric oxide. By relaxing blood arteries, nitric oxide enhances blood flow and reduces blood pressure. This action is comparable to that of several blood pressure medicines.

Lowering LDL Cholesterol Levels:

Research suggests that pomegranate juice regularly can lower blood levels of "bad" cholesterol, or LDL, which is cholesterol. Lowering LDL cholesterol levels is essential for heart health and may also help to sustain normal blood pressure.

ACE Blockers:

Pomegranate juice may naturally include angiotensin-converting enzyme (ACE) inhibitors, according to some research. One type of drug that is frequently recommended to treat hypertension is called ACE inhibitors. Pomegranate juice may help soften blood arteries and reduce blood pressure by suppressing ACE.

Studies on Blood Pressure Regulation:

Pomegranate juice's impact on blood pressure has been investigated in several clinical investigations. According to these research' encouraging findings, pomegranate juice drinking daily can significantly lower blood pressure readings, both diastolic and systolic.

Qualities of Natural Diuretics:

Additionally, pomegranate juice promotes greater urination due to its natural diuretic properties. By decreasing the amount of blood in the arteries and lowering blood pressure, this diuretic effect aids in the body's removal of extra salt and water.

Taking into Account

Pomegranate juice has potential as a natural blood pressure-lowering treatment, but it's important to take into account specific circumstances like allergies, drug interactions, and general diet. Before making big dietary changes, it's best to speak with a healthcare provider, particularly if there are any underlying medical issues or drugs to consider.

Pomegranate juice has many health benefits, including a high antioxidant content, the creation of nitric oxide, cholesterol-reducing effects, ACE inhibition, and natural diuretic effects. These attributes make it a promising natural therapy for decreasing blood pressure.

Individual reactions could differ, though, so speaking with a medical professional is essential to figuring out the best course of action for controlling hypertension.

CHAPTER EIGHT

Beet Juice

Beet juice's significant nutrient content—especially its high nitrate content—has made it a popular natural blood pressure-lowering treatment. Vegetables such as beets contain chemicals called nitrates, which are known to have a major impact on cardiovascular health.

Your body converts the nitrates in beets into nitric oxide when you drink beet juice. A chemical called nitric oxide aids in blood vessel dilatation, increasing blood flow and reducing blood pressure.

Here's how beet juice can help control high blood pressure:

Packed with Nitrates:

Nitrates are a naturally occurring compound that has vasodilator properties. They lower blood pressure by relaxing and widening blood arteries, which permits more blood to flow.

Enhances Endothelial Performance:

Nitric oxide, which is produced from the nitrates in beet juice, improves the endothelium (the inner lining of blood vessels) functionality. The endothelium must be in good health to control blood pressure.

Reduces Adverse Cholesterol:

According to studies, beet juice may help reduce high levels of low-density lipoprotein (LDL), which can lead to hypertension and heart disease.

Organic Diuretic:

Because of their inherent diuretic properties, beets help the body eliminate extra salt and water. This may contribute to lowering blood pressure by lowering blood volume.

Helps in Controlling Weight:

Beet juice can help with weight management because it is high in fiber and low in calories. Sustaining a healthy weight is crucial for blood pressure control.

Simple to Include:

It's simple to incorporate beet juice into your diet. It can be eaten on its own or blended into tasty and nourishing smoothies with other fruits and vegetables.

Study and Research:

Several investigations have been carried out to examine the potential advantages of beet juice in reducing blood pressure. Numerous studies have demonstrated beneficial outcomes in the decrease of both systolic and diastolic blood pressure, despite the possibility of individual responses differing.

Warnings and Points to Remember:

Although beet juice has potential benefits, it's crucial to remember that it may interfere with certain drugs or medical conditions. Because beets contain a significant amount of oxalate, people who have kidney difficulties or a history of kidney stones should exercise caution. Before making big dietary changes, it's always advisable to speak with a healthcare provider, particularly if you have underlying health problems.

Because of its high nitrate content, antioxidants, and other health benefits, beet juice is a promising natural blood pressure treatment. But it's crucial to include it in a varied, well-balanced diet, keeping in mind certain medical concerns, and speaking with a healthcare professional.

CHAPTER NINE

Prune Juice

A natural beverage made from dried plums, or prunes, prune juice is often drunk for its supposed blood pressure-lowering properties among other possible health advantages. Prunes may lower blood pressure, and there is some evidence to support this, but it is important to approach such statements cautiously and seek the opinion of a healthcare provider for specific recommendations.

Potassium, one of the several elements included in prune juice, is known to have a blood pressure-regulating effect. Elevated blood pressure can result from sodium levels in the body being out of balance, which potassium helps to regulate. Eating and drinking potassium-rich foods and drinks, including prune juice, may help to keep blood pressure levels in check.

An excellent source of dietary fiber is prune juice. In addition to being vital for heart health, fiber may also help to indirectly lower blood pressure. A diet rich in fiber helps lower cholesterol, assist control of weight, and enhance general cardiovascular health—all of which can have an impact on blood pressure.

It's important to remember that even though prune juice has healthy components, high blood pressure cannot be cured by it. An intricate disorder, high blood pressure is impacted by several variables, such as heredity, way of life, and general health. As a result, it's critical to manage blood pressure holistically, which may involve a healthy diet, frequent exercise, stress reduction, and, in certain situations, prescription medication from a medical professional.

Because of its high fiber and potassium content, prune that promotes can be included in a diet that promotes cardiovascular health. It shouldn't be considered a stand-alone treatment for decreasing blood pressure, though. For individualized advice on controlling high blood pressure and implementing healthy eating choices into your lifestyle, always seek the advice of a healthcare expert.

CHAPTER TEN

Blend of Berry Bliss

In addition to being a wonderful concoction of different berries, the Berry Bliss blend has become well-known for its possible health advantages, which include the potential to decrease blood pressure. Typically, this mixture contains berries that are high in antioxidants and important nutrients, such as blackberries, raspberries, strawberries, and blueberries.

Abundant in Antioxidants

The brilliant colors of berries are attributed to their high anthocyanin concentration or antioxidant content. These antioxidants support the body's defense against oxidative stress, which has been connected to several health problems, including elevated blood pressure.

Vasodilation
and Control of Blood Pressure:

Studies have been conducted on the substances found in berries, specifically flavonoids, and their propensity to induce vasodilation. The expansion of blood arteries, or vasodilation, has the potential to reduce blood pressure. The heart has to work less to move blood when the blood arteries are relaxed, which lowers blood pressure generally.

Abundant in Potassium

One important mineral that is necessary for controlling blood pressure is potassium. It assists in counteracting the impact of salt, which raises the risk of hypertension. Strawberries and blackberries in particular are excellent natural suppliers of potassium.

Its Anti-inflammatory Qualities

Chronic inflammation has been connected to several health issues, particularly high blood pressure.

Because they contain high concentrations of antioxidants as well as other bioactive substances, berries have anti-inflammatory characteristics that may help lower blood pressure by lowering inflammation.

Enhancing Vascular Performance:

According to research, eating berries daily may enhance blood vessel function. Maintaining optimum levels of blood pressure depends on the ability of healthy arteries to expand and constrict as needed. These arteries are more versatile.

Production of Nitric Oxide:

Additionally, berries may help the body produce nitric oxide. By facilitating blood channel relaxation, nitric oxide enhances blood flow and may lower blood pressure.

Maintaining Weight:

It is essential to maintain a healthy weight to control blood pressure. Because they are high in fiber and low in calories, berries are a healthy snack option for people trying to control their weight, which also helps to regulate blood pressure indirectly.

It's crucial to remember that, even though consuming Berry Bliss blend may help lower blood pressure, doing so should only be a small component of healthy living. Regular exercise, eating a balanced diet, controlling stress, and abstaining from extreme alcohol and tobacco use are all examples of this. Seeking individualized advice and support from a healthcare expert is always important if you have pre-existing medical problems or issues regarding your blood pressure.